COLLOIDAL SILVER

The Natural Antibiotic Alternative

By

Zane Baranowski, CN

IMPORTANT NOTICE:
This booklet is designed as an educational tool only. It is not meant to be used as a diagnosis, recommendation, or guarantee for any disease or result from using the information presented. Proper nutritional or medical attention should not be avoided or delayed when there is reason to seek professional help.

Published by Healing Wisdom Publications,
New York, NY 10023
ISBN #0-9647080-1-9

TABLE OF CONTENTS | PAGE

INTRODUCTION

Antibiotic-resistant germs are now considered epidemic in the United States, accounting for a growing number of serious infectious disorders. While most antibiotics disinfect about a half dozen or so germs, silver has been reported to disinfect hundreds. Most importantly, unlike conventional antibiotics, germs cannot build a resistance to the action of silver. A properly prepared colloid of silver is a special liquid preparation of this trace mineral that is extremely safe to use, even with children, without many of the negative side effects of prescription antibiotics.

When properly prepared, colloidal silver is a completely non-toxic, tasteless, internally and externally applicable, broad-spectrum germ fighter and disinfectant which can significantly reduce the length and severity of many bacterial infections. For these reasons and more, colloidal silver should prove to be one of the greatest discoveries in preventive, natural health care of all time.

WHAT IS A COLLOID?

The term colloid (KÖL' OID) refers to a substance that consists of ultra-fine particles that are suspended in a medium of different matter(i.e. a non-soluble mineral suspended in water). The particles in a colloid are typically 0.01 to 0.001 of a micron in diameter, or about four hundred thousandths to four millionths of an inch. Approximately one billion of these particles could fit into a cube four one hundredths of an inch in size. Diagram 1 shows the relative size of a colloid particle in microns (micron = μ).

The Russian scientist, S.S. Voyutsky, wrote that a colloidal system must have the following three characteristics: 1. It must be heterogeneous (meaning: consisting of dissimilar ingredients or constituents, like silver and water). 2. The system must be multiphasic (meaning: having more than one phase, i.e. solid/liquid, gas/liquid, etc). 3. The particles must be insoluble (meaning: does not dissolve) in the solution or suspension. Each one of these three characteristics interact with the others giving colloids their unique qualities. The fascinating thing about colloids is that they remain heterogeneous, multiphasic, and insoluble at different concentrations as long as a larger number, if not all of the particles, are within the range of sizes of colloids (ln to 100n, nanometers).

The particle size plays a major role in defining where a system falls. Below 1n (nanometer), the system will tend to be a molecular system. From 1n to 100n, the system falls within the constraints of a colloidal system. Coarse particles larger than 100n are usually found in systems that range from micro-heterogeneous systems, those that exhibit many of the same characteristics as colloids, to coarse suspensions - all of which are part of the dispersion system continuum. Microheterogeneous systems are a different color than that of a corresponding colloidal system. In a highly concentrated form, the color will tend to be more of a black color because the light passing through the suspension is blocked or reflected by the coarse particles. The coarse particles will also tend to fall out even if they have received an electrical charge like the smaller particles. Because gravity has more effect on a larger-sized particle, its effect is stronger than the repulsive forces of the electrical charge. Thus, the coarse particles will settle to the bottom of the container.

Elements have an affinity for each other on an atomic structure level. They are magnetically attracted to each other. They want to bond. The higher the concentration of the metal particles in a solution, the more likely the affinity attraction force of the metal particles for each other will bring them together and they will cling together in ever larger particles. Once they get to a certain largeness in size, they will precipitate out due to the action of gravity on them. In an ideal colloid the particles are small enough so that they will not cling together. Table A identifies these categories of solutions.

Diagram 1

Linear Magnification 1:10,000

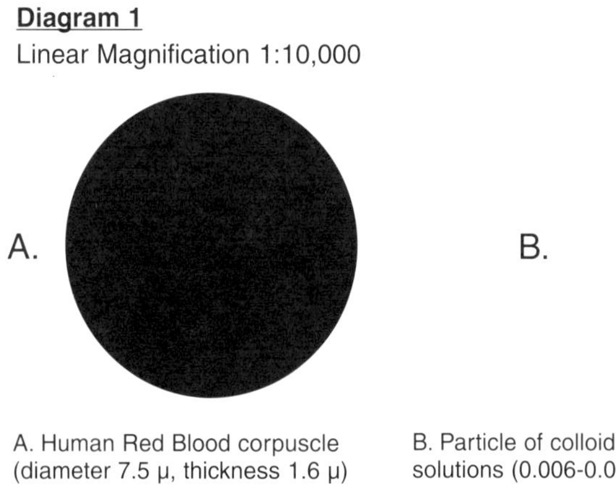

A. Human Red Blood corpuscle (diameter 7.5 μ, thickness 1.6 μ)

B. Particle of colloidal silver solutions (0.006-0.015 μ)

CURRENT STATUS

Colloidal silver is considered by the Food and Drug Administration to be a pre-1938 drug. The interpretation of this fact has created a lot of confusion in the marketplace, arising from a letter from the FDA dated 9/13/91 stating, "These products may continue to be marketed without submitted evidence of safety and effectiveness (required of all prescription drugs marketed after 1938) as long as they are advertised and labeled for the same use as in 1938 and as

TABLE A

0.1n	1n	10n	100n	1µ	10µ	100µ	1mm
Ultramicroscopic region				Microscopic region			
Particles show Brownian movement				No visible Brownian movement			
Particles pass through ordinary filter paper				Particles retained by filter paper			
Particles show increased solubility				Particles have ordinary solubility			
True solutions		Colloidal solutions		Emulsions and suspensions			
0.1n	1n	10n	100n	1µ	10µ	100µ	1mm

long as they are manufactured in the original manner." Many companies have construed this letter (which was officially reversed by another letter released from the FDA soon after) to grant the authority to make claims about colloidal silver's effectiveness against infectious disease. In fact, the current status of colloidal silver is that it can be manufactured and distributed, but no claims regarding effectiveness against disease can be made without going through the complicated and expensive drug approval process. It is one thing to say that colloidal silver has anti-bacterial properties; it is another thing to say that, because of these anti-bacterial properties, colloidal silver will 'cure' strep-throat or bronchitis.

METHODS OF PRODUCTION

Another source of confusion regarding colloidal silver is that a wide range of methods were used to manufacture colloids prior to 1938. These manufacturing approaches fall into five main groups. These include: (1) Grind (2) Wave (3) Liquid (4) Chemical and (5) Electrical. Table B portrays the various methods within the five groups colloids were manufactured. It also identifies the earliest recorded date when each method was employed.

TABLE B

Manufacturing Methods

Group	Method	Date
Grind	Ball Mill	1938
	Colloid Mill	1920
	Disk/China Mill	1924
	Aerodispersion Mill	1927
Wave	Ultrasonic	1921
	Radiant Energy	1910
Liquid	Homogenizers	1930
	Prolonged boiling in water	1910
	Mercury Vapor condensed on water	1920
Chemical	Chemical Action	1860
Electrical	Electrical Arts	1924
	Cathode atomization	1926
	Vacuum evaporation	1927
	Electrosputtering	1898

Of these five manufacturing processes, the grind process and the electro-colloidal process were primarily used to manufacture colloidal silver. Today, the FDA still allows both manufacturing techniques to be used. However, of these two methods the electro-colloidal manufacturing process is generally considered to be far superior. With the grind method the particles of silver are usually no finer than four one-thousands of an inch. They may or may not be electrically charged. The size of the silver particle is so large compared to the possible charge, that the repelling forces would not be strong enough to offset the pull of gravity on the particles, which will tend to settle to the bottom of the solution, producing a less effective product.

To offset this settling problem, some manufacturers add a "stabilizer" (usually a protein) to make the solution more viscous and keep them suspended for a longer period of time. The silver particles will still eventually settle to the bottom. The container will have to be shaken to re-disperse the particles. However, stabilizers tend to block the beneficial effects of the silver particles.

Other procedures used in producing colloidal silver that involve a simple mixture of metal and liquid (grind process) cannot possess as much potential as electro-colloids and are therefore of questionable value. The proper electrical process allows silver particles to be drawn off the ingot that are much smaller than four one-thousandths of an inch diameter. If the silver particles are within the range of four one-hundred-thousands to four one-millionths of an inch in diameter, and are uniformly charged, a stabilizer is not required to keep the particles suspended. The repelling magnetic force will offset the pull of gravity on the particles, which are animated by "Brownian Movement", and remain in suspension in a liquid medium almost indefinitely, their stability depending on the size of the particles, the medium used and the manufacturing process employed.

EARLY USES OF COLLOIDAL SILVER

Another source of confusion regarding the current use of colloidal silver has been the lack of information about which form was originally used. It is known that, prior to 1938, colloidal silver was administered in just about every way that modern drugs are administered: intravenous and intra-muscular injection, throat gargle, douche, oral use, topical administration, and as eye drops. What is not well known is the precise form of colloidal silver used, its concentration, and precise dosage for effective results.

Robert J. Hartman in 1939 writes, "Aqueous metallic silver suspensions...are used extensively as a gargle and, in genito-urinary diseases, as a douche, or irrigant for inflamed mucous membranes. Certain of these colloidal suspensions are prepared that can be injected intravenously or intramuscularly... metallic silver in colloidal suspension...yield silver ions in such a quantity as to have a detrimental effect on microorganisms but slowly enough not to be irritating to the tissues. The colloidal silver particles provide a continuous source of these ions, yet the particles are not absorbed by the body tissue taken en masse in true solution by the body fluids. Consequently, colloidal silver can be applied directly to delicate mucous membranes, such as those in the eye, with no irritation and with beneficial results... The colloidal particles diffuse gradually throughout the blood and give prolonged therapeutic action."

On the other end of the dispersion continuum, Kopaczewski suggests that the size of particles in suspensions has an impact on effectiveness. He writes, "Two facts seem to support the view that the antiseptic effect is attributable to the colloidal state: (1) Only finely dispersed colloids have an antiseptic effect. This would indicate that the physical condition of the colloid is of importance. It was moreover shown by conductivity measurements and qualitative analysis that the amount of dissolved silver and silver oxide in coarse grained solution on one hand and in fine-grained on the other, is by no means equal, and that it is considerably higher in the latter. (2) It was observed by V. Henri that when the inter-micellar fluid of a fine grained colloidal solution was separated from the micelles (larger particles) by filtration, and (the micelles) added to a culture, it produced no antiseptic effect. This led Henri to the conclusion that the antiseptic effect is an inherent quality of the colloidal state."

Alfred Searle, in 1919, after describing silver and other metal colloids, writes, "The germicidal action of certain metals in the colloidal state having been demonstrated, it only remained to apply them to the human subject, and this has been done in a large number of cases with astonishingly successful results. It is not suggested that colloidal metal solutions should replace the customary disinfectants for sterilizing excreta, vessels of various kinds and for other general purposes (ed. At the time it was too expensive for such use), but for internal administration, either orally or hypodermically, they have the advantage of being rapidly fatal to the parasites both bacterial and otherwise without any toxic action on the host. "

Searle further states that "Colloidal silver solution is quite stable even in the presence of salts and of the normal constituents of the blood. Its destructive action on toxins is very marked, so that it will protect rabbits from ten times the lethal dose of tetanic (from tetanus) or diphtheric (from diphtheria) toxin."

Regarding the use of metallic colloids in medicine, Dr. Leonard Keene Hirschberg writes, "Speaking generally, the colloidal metals are especially remarkable for their beneficial action in infective states of blood poisoning by germs. This action has been shown to be due to their stimulating influence and to their destructive effects on micro-organisms and their toxins as shown by the immediate fall of temperature, and the subsidence of the constitutional symptoms of intoxication.

C. E. A. MacLeod reports colloidal silver being used with marked success in the following cases: "Septic and follicular tonsillitis, Vincent's angina, phlyctenular conjunctivitis, gonorrheal conjunctivitis, spring catarrh, impetigo (contagious acne of face and body), septic ulcers of legs, ringworm of body, tinea versicolor, soft sores, suppurative appendicitis after operation (the wounds cleaned rapidly), pustular eczema of scalp and pubes, chronic eczema of meatus of ear with recurrent boils, and also chronic eczema of anterior nares, offensive discharge in case of chronic suppuration in otitis media, bromidrosis of feet, axilla and blind boils of neck. By injection: gonorrhoea and chronic cystitis (local), boils, epididymitis."

Sir James Cantlie found it very effective, "in cases of sprue, dysentery, and intestinal troubles."

A. Legge Roe regarded, "stable colloidal silver as a most useful preparation in ophthalmic practice, and particularly in cases of gonorrheal ophthalmia, purulent ophthalmia of infants, infected ulcers of the cornea and hypopyon ulcer (tapping of the interior chamber and cautery, and other operative procedures being now rarely required, whilst if perforation does occur it is smaller and more manageable), interstitial keratitis, blepharitis, dacryocystitis, and burns and other wounds of the cornea. According to this authority, if the great chemosis which usually accompanies the use of silver were adopted in every case of purulent ophthalmia of infants 'there would be no such thing as impaired sight or blindness from this cause.' He has had many cases of interstitial keratitis in adults, in which the complete opacity of the cornea has become absolutely clear in from three to five months, and anyone who has had much experience of this disease in adults knows how often permanent impairment of sight results, and how long the treatment used to last, especially if irritants had been used prior to colloidal treatment...the colloidal solution is dropped in three times a day, the eye being kept closed afterwards for five minutes."

Professor Wolfgang Ostwald noted, "All life processes....take place in a colloidal system, and that is true both of the normal fluids and secretions of the organism and of the bacterial toxins, as well as, in large measure, of the reactions which confer immunity." Based on that premise, Alfred Searle writes that, "Fortunately, the recognition of bacteria and their products as essentially colloidal in character has greatly facilitated the study of disinfection. It is now realized that - disregarding the fact that bacteria are alive - they may - owing to their colloidal character and that of the toxins and some other substances they produce - be destroyed by substances which bear an electrical charge opposite to that of the bacteria or their colloidal products... The great advantage of dealing with germs as colloids lies in the fact that the agents used for their coagulation and consequent destruction are not necessarily poisonous, an advantage which becomes of utmost importance when it is desired to destroy the bacteria in corpore villi....By converting the metal into the colloidal state it may be applied in a much more concentrated form and with correspondingly better results."

An important advantage of using colloidal silver is that it has no recorded side effects. Also, Searle found that colloidal silver does not stain the skin, unlike certain pharmaceutical preparations of silver that do produce strong stains.

REDISCOVERING THE UNIVERSAL ANTIMICROBIAL

Silver is one of the most universal antibiotic substances. When administered in the colloidal form, it is for all practical purposes, non-toxic. Silver has been proven to be useful against hundreds of infectious conditions. Although the exact mechanism for the proven antimicrobial effects of silver is unknown, the most accepted theory is that silver disables the specific enzyme that many forms of bacteria, viruses and fungi utilize for their metabolism.

Prior to 1938, colloidal silver was considered to be one of the mainstays of antibiotic treatment. At that time it was considered to be quite "high-tech", but compared to today's colloidal silver solutions, it was technically inferior. In the early 1900's the silver particle never reached its optimum therapeutic ultra-microscopic size. Nevertheless, such prestigious medical journals as The Lancet (1914) published the results of scientific studies examining the successful use of colloidal silver. For a period of time the use of silver as a medicine fell out of favor. One reason was Argyria - a skin discoloration that results when hundreds of times the proper amount of silver compounds are injected or taken orally, and silver is deposited under the skin, giving a harmless but unsightly gray coloration.

The comeback of silver in medicine began in the 1970's. The late Dr. Carl Moyer, chairman of Washington University's Department of Surgery, received a grant to develop better treatments for burn victims. Dr. Margraf, as the chief biochemist, worked with Dr. Moyer and other surgeons to find an antiseptic strong enough, yet safe to use over large areas of the body. Dr. Margraf reviewed 22 antiseptic compounds and found drawbacks in all of them. "Mercury, for example, is an excellent antiseptic but toxic," he comments. "Popular antiseptics....can be used over small areas only." Furthermore, disease organisms can become resistant to antibiotics, triggering a dangerous super-infection. "These compounds are also ineffective against a number of harmful bacteria, including the biggest killer in burn cases - a greenish-blue bacterium called Pseudomonas aeruginosa. It almost always shows up in burns, releasing a poison."

Reviewing medical literature, Dr. Margraf found repeated references to silver. It was described as a catalyst that disables the enzymes microorganisms depend on to "breathe." Consequently, they die. Therefore, Dr. Margraf decided to use the best known compound of silver: silver nitrate. Concentrated silver nitrate was corrosive and painful. So he diluted the silver nitrate to a .5 percent solution and found that it killed the Pseudomonas aeruginosa bacteria and permitted wounds to heal. Resistant strains did not appear. Silver nitrate, however, was far from ideal. It disturbed the balance of body salts, was thick and cumbersome to use and stained everything it touched. Dr. Margraf searched for other preparations of silver. As a result of these efforts, hundreds of important new medical uses for silver were found. Medical journal reports from the early 1900's demonstrated a properly prepared colloid of silver was the only form of silver solution that was not deposited under the skin, no matter how many times the proper amount was administered. There were still skeptics. Some of the negative reaction that colloidal silver received in the early 1900's, "was due to a premature supply of improperly prepared and unstable colloids... Shortly after the definite recognition of the colloidal nature of the chief body fluids was effected, the enormous possibilities which might result from the application of colloidal disinfectants and medicines were rapidly recognized....A number of colloidal substances were placed on the market...in this country and elsewhere....It was soon found, however, that most of these preparations rapidly deteriorated in value: some of them were so unstable that they contained no active colloid at the time when they were used."

N.R. Thompson recognized that, "To primitive life forms, oligodynamic silver is as toxic as the most powerful chemical disinfectants and this, coupled with its relative harmlessness to animate life (i.e. mammals), gives it great potential as a disinfectant."

Based on laboratory tests with colloidal silver, destructive bacteria, virus, and fungus organisms are killed within minutes of contact. Larry C. Ford, M.D. of the Department of Obstetrics and Gynecology, UCLA School of Medicine, Center For The Health Sciences reported in a letter dated November 1, 1988, "I tested them (the silver solutions) using standard antimicrobial tests for disinfectants. The silver solutions were antibacterial for concentrations of 10^5 organisms per ml. of Streptococcus Pyogenes, Staphylococcus Aureus, Neisseria Gonorrhea, Gardnerella Vaginalis, Salmonella Typhi, and other enteric pathogens, and fungicidal for Candida Albicans, Candida Globata, and M. Furfur."

Jim Powell reported in a Science Digest article March, 1978, titled, "Our Mightiest Germ Fighter", "Thanks to eye-opening research, silver is emerging as a wonder of modern medicine. An antibiotic kills perhaps a half-dozen different disease organisms, but silver kills some 650. Resistant strains fail to develop. Moreover, silver is virtually non-toxic." Dr. Harry Margraf of St. Louis concluded "Silver is the best all around germ-fighter we have."

The future of colloidal silver is bright. Hopefully with today's technological advances, we can avoid the past mistakes and benefit from its wide range of advantages to prevent and treat infectious disorders.

VISUAL QUALITIES

One indicator of the quality of colloidal silver is its color. As the size of each silver particle gets larger, the color of the suspension ranges from yellow (best) to brown, to red, to gray, to black (inferior). The increasing size of the particles also reflects a proportionate decrease in quality of the product. Colloids of silver that are produced using the electro-colloidal method are a different color than the grind or chemical method forms of colloidal silver. That rule generally applies, except in the case of some brands that use an artificial yellow dye to falsify the proper color. Color variance also depends on concentration, stabilizers, and the presence or absence of other trace elements. The ideal form of colloidal silver will be almost colorless or have a very light yellow color.

Besides buying from a reputable company and visually checking the color of the product, another quick way to see if a solution contains colloids is by observing the Faraday-Tyndall cone effect. When a sharp and intense beam of light passes through a colloid solution, the path of the light will appear to be turbid. The path of the light is also altered. The path of the light will form a cone shape within the solution. The best way to observe this is to take a test tube of colloidal silver into a dark room and shine a very bright flash light through it. Colloids will appear to be milky. (Note: a discussion can be found in Jirgensons and Straumanis' book titled "A Short Textbook of Colloid Chemistry;" New York: John Wiley & Sons, Inc; London: Pergamon Press Ltd.; 1954.)

BEST COLLOIDAL SILVER

Within the last few years, a number of colloidal silver products have appeared on the market, confusing consumers. The best way to determine if a product is a true colloid of silver is to examine the ingredients. If it contains a stabilizer, or listed trace elements other than silver, the product may not be suitable. If the product requires refrigeration, it may contain some other ingredient that might spoil at room temperature.

The highest quality colloidal silver is produced by the electro-colloidal/non-chemical method. The silver particles and water have been completely "colloided" and evenly dispersed and held in suspension by an electrical current sent through the combination. This process is the only known method to create a truly homogeneous (evenly distributed) solution, containing super-fine silver particles in the range of 0.005 - 0.015 microns in diameter, suspended in water, without the need of any chemical, stabilizer, dye, or other ingredient. There is very little or no visible accumulation of silver particles either in the solution or settled on the bottom. The best products will contain the largest number of particles from the smallest total amount of silver. (Note: an artificial electrical charge applied to any element, including silver, cannot be held infinitely - like a battery, its charge will dissipate. Therefore, electro-colloidal silver cannot be expected to have infinite shelf-life; some 'fallout' may occur in any non-stabilized product over an extended period of time.)

SAFETY AND EFFECTIVENESS

Specific documentation on the optimum potency or dosage for effective use is sparse. This has led to a wide range of products of vary - ing potencies - all claiming to be the best. According to N.R. Thompson of Runcorn Health Laboratory in England, the concentration of silver necessary to sterilize water contaminated with pathogenic bacteria is between 40-200 gamma, or .04 to .2ppm (1 ppm = 1000 gamma). In 1940 and 1966, respectively, R.A. Kehoe and I.H. Tipton reported that under normal circumstances the average daily diet will yield approximately 50mcg to 100mcg of silver. (Note: The reduction of silver in the average diet, due to commercial farming techniques, is similar to what has happened with other trace minerals including chromium, zinc and selenium - that are now known to be essential for good health. This reduction may play a role in the worldwide epidemic of chronic infections.)

Therefore, it seems logical that a concentration of 3 to 5 ppm, yielding 15 mcg to 25 mcg of silver per teaspoon, will be a sufficient concentration to be both effective and safe to consume on a regular, daily basis. A 4 oz. container of colloidal silver at a concentration of 3 ppm will contain approximately 355 mcg of total silver - well below any reported toxicity level of orally consumed silver - even if several ounces were consumed on a daily basis for several years. Higher concentrations above 5 ppm, or about 591 mcg of total silver in a 4 oz container, may cause silver build-up in the system and are not necessarily more effective. For example, a 25 ppm solution would yield 2.96 mg (2,960 mcg), a 500 ppm solution would yield 59 mg (59,000 mcg), a 5,000 ppm solution would yield 590 mg (590,000 mcg)! Any product containing higher concentrations, for example having higher levels than what could be found in the average daily diet, should definitely be taken with caution, only during a time of need and certainly not for extended periods.

The statement 'less is more' is often made when referring to colloidal silver and colloidal technology in general. What this means is that the number of silver particles determines the quality and effectiveness of colloidal silver, NOT simply the concentration. The term 'ppm' or 'parts per million' is confusing because it is not referring to the number of parts or particles, it is actually a different way to express total weight or total amount of silver. Since a colloidal product can have particles ranging in size from 1n to100n, it is difficult to judge the quality of a product by simply knowing the ppm. For example, a product with a concentration of 5 ppm with an average particle size of 5n would actually have more silver particles than another product of 25ppm with an average size of 50n and thus be safer and more effective.

Stability, especially long-term, is another important aspect of colloidal silver products. To avoid "fall out", some companies add a protein or chemical stabilizer, allowing a higher concentration of silver with a greater level of stability. The downside is that most stabilizers bond to and therefore reduce the antimicrobial effect of silver. Such products contain higher levels of total silver to compensate, and should be taken with caution because in all documented cases of silver toxicity, called Argyria (the permanent discoloration of the skin due to silver deposits), the product in question contained high concentrations of silver compounded with stabilizers such as silver nitrate or silver acetate. Argyria has never been reported from pure electro-colloidal silver free of protein or other stabilizers.

Another advantage of correctly manufactured colloidal silver is that, with a particle size well below 1 micron (.015 to .001), a 3 to 5ppm concentration of colloidal silver is unlikely to affect friendly intestinal bacteria. When taken orally, sublingual absorption in the mouth directly into the bloodstream should occur before the silver particles have the opportunity to migrate into the small or large intestine where intestinal bacteria normally dominate. However, in the case of a known intestinal infection, enemas or colonics of colloidal silver could be utilized to directly expose the infection to the sterilizing benefit of colloidal silver. Consumption of colloidal silver on a daily basis would significantly reduce the incidence of infection. The ability to do this safely could be a powerful preventive health measure to enhance the lives of millions of people susceptible to chronic infections. This is an opportunity only offered by properly prepared electrocolloidal silver that contains 99.9999% pure silver with no binding agents, stabilizers or proteins.

MODERN DAY USES

Although reports on the use of colloidal silver have spanned the past 100 years, research relating to its recent use is limited. However, through a growing number of physicians, dentists, veterinarians, nutritionists and satisfied users, information regarding the modern day uses of colloidal silver is mounting.

This information in no way 'proves' colloidal silver 'cures' infectious disorders or disease, and this claim should not be made by any reputable colloidal silver manufacturer. However it is proven that colloidal silver does have tremendous antimicrobial power; the history of safe and successful colloidal silver use is extensive, and the number of current health professionals and individuals that successfully utilize colloidal silver to reduce the length and severity of infectious disorders is growing exponentially.

TABLE C
Colloidal Silver Applications

Systemic Internal Infections	**Localized External Infections**
flu/fevers	eyes & ears
herpes	ore throat
hepatitis	abcesses/dental
epstein-barr	nasal/sinus
bronchitis	poison oak & rashes
pneumonia	burns, cuts & bites
yeast/vaginal	ahtletes foot or groin

Table C lists some, but certainly not all, of the helpful uses of colloidal silver for modern day problems. (Note: colloidal silver is also applicable for infectious disorders relating to pets including cats, dogs, birds and horses.)

The amount and method of application of colloidal silver for many of these conditions depends primarily upon whether the infection is localized, as in an ear, eye or sinus infection, or systemic, as in flu, fever or hepatitis.

Localized infections are generally easier to treat than systemic infections because the colloidal silver can be applied directly to the infectious organism (i.e. poured into the ear canal, dropped into the eye, sprayed into the nose, vaporized into the lung). With systemic infections, including fevers, herpes and hepatitis, the amount of silver used and the length of time for treatment will have to be determined by the severity of infection, age, weight and overall health. Users will do best to rely on labels combined with information from other sources with direct clinical experience.

Overall, it seems that the effective and safe use of colloidal silver in the treatment of dozens of common infectious disorders is only limited by the imagination and creativity of those afflicted.

Bibliography, References & Resources

Higher Education Library Publishers (H.E.L.P. ful news), Colloidal Silver - A Closer Look., Vol. 9- 11.

Alexander, J. Colloid Chemistry. Van Nostrand Co.: New York, N.Y. 1924, p. 33.

Freundlich, H. The Elements of Colloidal Chemistry, translated by G. Barger. Methuen & Co. LTD.: London, 1925, p. 131.

Freundlich, H. Colloid & Capillary Chemistry, Translated by H. S. Hatfield. E.P. Dutton and Company, Inc.: New York, 1922, p. 740-742.

Voyutsky, S. Colloid Chemistry, translated by N. Bobrov. Mir Publishers: Moscow, 1978, p.21.

Goddard, E. D., "Colloid," The World Book Encyclopedia. World Book Inc.: Chicago, 1985,Vol. 4, p. 623.

South, James, Electro-Colloidal Silver: The Amazing Anti-Microbial, Lecture given at Natural Products Expo West, Anaheim, 3/10/94. Available from Teamwork Marketing, PO Box 916, San Anselmo, CA 94979.

Hauser, E. A. Colloidal Phenomena, an Introduction to the Science of Colloids. McGraw-Hill Book Company, Inc.: New York, 1939, pp. 59 - 73.

Brentano, L. MD, Margraf, H., Monafo, W.W. MD and Moyer, C.A. MD. Antibacterial Efficacy of a Colloidal Silver Complex. Surgical Forum, Vol. 17, 1966, pp. 76 - 78.

Hirschberg, Dr. Leonard Keene "Electrical Colloids" from an article out of Johns Hopkins Hospital.

Kopaczewski, W. "The Pharmacodynamics of Colloids," Colloid chemistry theoretical and applied, ed. J. Alexander, The Book Department, The Chemical Catalog Company, Inc.: New York, Vol. 2, 1928, p. 962.

Bechhold, H. Colloids in Biology and Medicine, translated by J. G. M. Bullow. D. Van Nostrand Company: New York, 1919, p. 359.

Hartman, R.J. Colloid Chemistry. Houghton Mifflin Company: Boston, 1939, p. 536.

Searle, A.B. The Use of Colloids in Health and Disease. E.P. Dutton & Company: New York, 1919, p. 75.

Jim Powell, "Our Mightiest Germ Fighter", Science Digest, March 1978, p. 59-60.

Kehoe RA et al, 1940. J. Nutr. 19. 579.

Tipton IH et al,1966. Health Physics 12. 1683.

N.R. Thompson. Comprehensive Inorganic Chemistry. Volume 5, chapter 28, Pergamon Press, Elmsford, New York. 1973.

W.R Hill, MD and D.M. Pillsbury, MA, MD. Argyria-The Pharmacology of Silver. Williams & Wilkins Company, 1939.

East BW et al, Silver retention, Total Body Silver and Tissue Silver concentrations in argyria associated with exposure to an anti-smoking remedy containing silver acetate. Clinical and Experimental Dermatology. 1980. 5, 305-311.

Larry C. Ford, MD, Department of Obstetrics and Gynecology, UCLA School of Medicine, Center For The Health Sciences. 1988 letter available from Teamwork Marketing, PO Box 916, San Anselmo, CA 94979.

Recent articles have described silver being used to treat:

Adenovirus 5,23	Aspergillus Niger 18
Bacillius Typhosus 21	Bovine Rotavirus 23
Candida Albicans 18	Entamoeba Histolytica (Cysts)24
Escherichia Coli1 7,18,21	Legionella Pneumophila 17
Poliovirus 1 (Sabin Strain) 23	Pseudomonas Aeruginosa 17,18
Salmonella 22	Spore-Forming Bacteria 24
Staphylococcus Aureus 17	Streptococcus Faecalis 17
Vegetative B. Cereus Cells 24	

COLLOIDAL SILVER USES BEFORE 1938

Table D lists some of the (pre-1938) documented uses of silver, including the colloidal form, for the treatment of various conditions and pathogens. This list in no way should be construed or relied upon as medical advice. Always consult your health care professional if a serious condition exists.

TABLE D COLLOIDAL SILVER ITS USES BEFORE 1938

Numbers refer to Bibliographic Footnotes

Use	Ref.	Use	Ref.
Appendicitis (post-op)	3	Gonorrhoeal Conjunctivitis	10
B. Coli	2	Hypopyon Ulcer	13
B. Dysenteria	2	Infantile Disease	16
Anthrax Bacilli	2,3	Inflammatory Rheumatism	3
Axillae and Blind Boils of the Neck	10	Interstitial Keratitis	13
B. Coli Communis	7	Ophthalmology	12
B. Pyocaneus	2	Para-Typhoid	3
Bacillary Dysentery	4	Perineal Eczemal	2
Blepharitis	3	Phlegmons	3,31, 32
Bromidrosis in Axille	2	Pneumococci	2
Burns and Wounds of the Corneal	3	Puerperal Septicemia	15
Chronic Cystitis	10	Pustular Eczema of Scalp	10
Chronic Eczema of Meatus of Ear	10	Phlyctenular Conjunctivitis	10
Cystitis	8	Pruritis Ani	12
Dermatitis suggestive of Toxaemia	4	Purulent Opthalmia of Infants	13
Diptheria	3	Pyorrhoea Alveolaris (Rigg's Disease)	8
Epiditymitis	10	Quinsies	3
Eustachian Tubes (potency restored)	8	Rhinitis	9
Furunculosis	3	Scarlatina	3
Gonorrhoea	10	Septic Tonsillitis	10
Gonorrhoea Opthalmial	3	Septicemia	5, 8
Hemorrhoids	2	Soft Sores	10
Impetigo	10	Sprue	6
Infected Ulcers of the Cornea	3	Staphylococcus Pyogenea	7
Influenza	11	Staphylococcus Pyogens Aureus	2
Intestinal Troubles	6	Subdues Inflammation	12
Leucorrhoea	8	Tinea Versicolor	10
Nasal Catarrh	5	Tyhpoid	3
Edematous enlargement of Turbinates without True Hyperplasia	9	Ulcerative Urticaria	4
Offensive Discharge of Chronic Supporation in Otitis Media	10	Valsava's Inflammation	3
B. Tuberculosis	7	Vorticella	1
Bladder Irritation	12	Whooping Cough	8
Boils	10	Ringworm of the body	10
Bromidrosis in Feet	10	Sepsis	16
Cerebro-spinal Meningitis	3, 9	Septic Ulcers of the legs	10
Chronic Eczema of Anterior Nares	10	Shingles	8
Colitis	4	Spring Catarrh	10
Dacrocystitis	13	Staphyloclysin (inhibits)	2
Diarrhea	4	Staphylococcus Pyogens Albus	2
Dysentery	3, 6	Streptococci	7
Enlarged Prostate	12	Suppurative Appenclicitis (post-op)	10
Erysipelas	3	Tonsillitis	8
Follicular Tonsilittis	10	Typhoid Bacillus	14
Gonococcus	7	Urticaria suggestive of Toxaemia	12
		Vincent's Angina	10
		Warts	2

Bibliographic Footnotes for Diseases

1. Bechhold, H. Colloids in biology and medicine, translated by J. G. M. Bulloow. D. Van Nostrand Company: New York, 1919, p. 367.

2. Ibid., p. 368.

3. Ibid., p. 376.

4. Searle, A. B. The use of colloids in health and disease. (Quoting from the British Medical Journal, May 12, 1917) E. P. Dutton & Company: New York, 1919, p. 82.

5. Ibid., (Quoting from the British Medical Journal, Jan. 15, 1917) p. 83.

6. Ibid., (Quoting Sir James Cantlie in the British Medical Journal, Nov. 15, 1913) p. 83.

7. Ibid., (Quoting Henry Crookes) p. 70.

8. Ibid., (Quoting J. Mark Hovell in the British Medical Journal, Dec. 15, 1917) p. 86.

9. Ibid., (Quoting B. Seymour Jones) p. 86.

10. Ibid., (Quoting C. E. A. MacLeod in Lancet, Feb. 3, 1912) p. 83.

11. Ibid., (Quoting J. MacMunn in the British Medical Journal, 1917, I, 685) p. 86.

12. Ibid., (Quoting Sir Malcolm Morris in the British Medical Journal, May 12, 1917) p. 85.

13. Ibid., (Quoting A. Legge Roe in the British Medical Journal, Jan. 16, 1915) p. 83.

14. Ibid., (Quoting W. J. Simpson in Lancet, Dec. 12, 1914) pp. 71-72.

15. Ibid., (Quoting T. H. Anderson Wells in Lancet, Feb. 16, 1918) p. 85.

16. Index-catalogue of the Library of the Surgeon General's Office United States Army. United States Government Printing Office: Washington, v. IX, 1913, p. 628.

17. Moyasar, T. Y.; Landeen, L. K.; Messina, M. C.; Kutz, S. M.; Schulze, R.; and Gerba, C. P. Disinfection of bacteria in water systems by using electrolytically generated copper, silver and reduced levels of free chlorine. Found in Canadian Journal of Microbiology. The National Research Council of Canada: Ottawa, Ont., Canada, 1919, pp. 109-116.

18. Simonetti, N.; Simonetti, G.; Bougnol, F.; and Scalzo, M. Electrochemical AG+ for preservative use. Article found in Applied and Environmental Microbiology. American Society for Microbiology: Washington, v. 58, 12, 1992,pp. 3834-3836.

19. Slawson, R M.; Van Dyke, M. I.; Lee, H.; and Trevors, J. T. Germanium and silver resistance, accumulation, and toxicity in microorganisms. Article found in Plasmid. Academic Press, Inc.: San Diego, v.27, 1, 1992,73-79.

20. Thurman, R B. and Gerba, C. P. The molecular mechanisms of copper and silver ion disinfection of bacteria and viruses. A paper presented in the First International Conference on Gold and Silver in Medicine. The Silver Institute: Washington, v. 18, 4, 1989, p. 295.

21. Ibid., p. 299.

22. Ibid., p. 300.

23. Ibid., p. 301.

24. Ibid., p. 302.

0 94717 27945 3

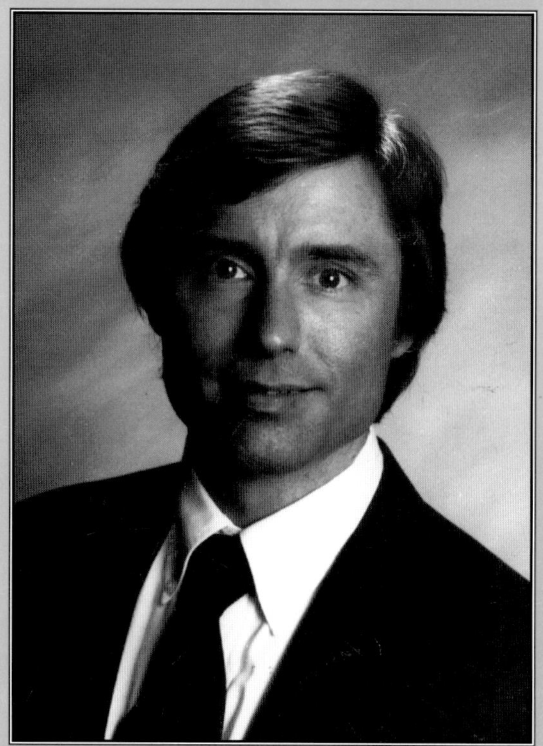

Zane Baranowski, CN is a certified nutritionist from the National Institute of Nutritional Education in Aurora, Colorado. He has been a nutritional research and product development consultant to health food supplement manufacturers and distributors for over 10 years.

His specific area of focus is the prevention and treatment of degenerative conditions with diet